# LOSE  WEIGHT  AND  STAY  BUSY:
## Tips for Effective Weight Loss

By     ESTHER M KOCH

Table of Content

<u>The Ongoing Journey of Health and Wellness after Weight Loss therapy</u>.

# PREFACE

Losing weight can be a challenging journey, especially when you have a busy schedule. It can be challenging to find the time and energy to exercise regularly and prepare healthy meals. However, with the right mindset and a few simple tips, you can achieve your weight loss goals while still managing your busy lifestyle.

Read , Meditate and Practice these simple tips on weight loss. Pray and believe in every step you follow. You are blessed with regenerational power creating again deformed systems. Just say I CAN.

This book, "Lose Weight and Stay Busy: Tips for Effective Weight Loss," is designed to provide you with practical advice and strategies to help you lose weight and maintain a healthy lifestyle, even when you have a full plate.

In this book, you will find a variety of tips and techniques that are specifically tailored to fit into a busy schedule. From simple lifestyle changes to quick and effective workouts, you will learn how to make the most of your time and achieve your weight loss goals without sacrificing your other responsibilities.

Whether you are a working professional, a busy parent, or simply someone with a lot on your plate, this book will provide you with the guidance you need to lose weight and stay busy. With the right mindset, dedication, and support, you can achieve your weight loss goals and live a healthier, more fulfilling life.

## INTRODUCTION

Starting a healthier weight is a personal commitment towards achieving a healthier body weight and improving overall wellness. This journey is not a quick fix but a gradual process that requires dedication, patience, and consistency.

The first step in this journey is setting realistic goals. It is important to identify how much weight needs to be lost, and then break that down into achievable goals. This approach makes the process less overwhelming and more manageable. Additionally, setting specific targets will help track progress and stay motivated.

A balanced diet is an essential part of achieving a healthier weight. This involves consuming a variety of nutrient-dense foods such as fruits, vegetables, whole grains, lean protein, and healthy fats. Avoiding processed and high-calorie foods, and reducing portion sizes can also be helpful. Moreover, keeping a food diary or using a food tracking app can provide valuable insights into eating habits and help make better food choices.

Physical activity is also crucial in achieving a healthier weight. Engaging in regular exercise, such as walking, jogging, swimming, or cycling, can help burn calories and increase metabolism. It is important to start with realistic exercise goals and gradually increase the intensity and duration of physical activity.

In addition to diet and exercise, maintaining a healthy lifestyle is essential. Adequate sleep, reducing stress, and avoiding unhealthy habits such as smoking and excessive drinking can have a positive impact on overall health and weight.

It is important to remember that the journey to a healthier weight is not about perfection but progress. Celebrating small successes and learning from setbacks can help maintain motivation and stay on track. Seeking support from friends, family, or a healthcare professional can also be beneficial.In conclusion, the journey to a healthier weight is a personal commitment towards achieving better health and well-being. It requires a balanced diet, regular physical activity, and a healthy lifestyle. It may not be easy, but with dedication, patience, and consistency, it is achievable.

## The Importance of Staying Busy in Weight Loss

Staying busy is an important aspect of weight loss that is often overlooked. Many people believe that simply changing their diet and exercising regularly is enough to achieve their weight loss goals. However, keeping yourself occupied and engaged in activities that you enjoy can be a powerful tool for achieving long-term weight loss success.

Firstly, staying busy helps to prevent boredom and the temptation to overeat. When people are idle or have too much free time, they often turn to food for entertainment or comfort. However, staying busy with productive activities such as work, hobbies, or social events can help distract from food cravings and reduce the likelihood of overeating.

Secondly, staying busy can increase physical activity levels. Sitting idle or watching TV for long periods of time can lead to a sedentary lifestyle, which can contribute to weight gain. On the other hand, engaging in active hobbies such as hiking, dancing, or sports can provide a fun and effective way to burn calories and increase fitness levels.

Thirdly, staying busy can help to reduce stress levels, which is crucial for weight loss success. Stress can trigger overeating, particularly of high-calorie comfort foods. Engaging in activities that promote relaxation and reduce stress such as yoga, meditation, or taking a bath can help to prevent emotional eating.

Finally, staying busy can improve overall mental health, which can contribute to weight loss success. Depression, anxiety, and other mental health issues can contribute to overeating and unhealthy food choices. Engaging in activities that promote positive emotions such as volunteering, spending time with loved ones, or pursuing personal goals can boost self-esteem and promote a positive mindset.

In conclusion, staying busy is a vital component of successful weight loss. It can prevent boredom and overeating, increase physical activity levels, reduce stress, and improve mental health. By incorporating enjoyable and productive activities into your daily routine, you can stay motivated, reduce cravings, and achieve your weight loss goals.

Losing weight can be challenging, especially if you lead a busy lifestyle. However, incorporating physical activity into your daily routine can help you shed those extra pounds and maintain a healthy weight. In this article, we will discuss some effective strategies for incorporating physical activity into your busy lifestyle to help you lose weight and stay fit.

Schedule Your Workout Time:

One of the most important strategies for incorporating physical activity into your busy lifestyle is to schedule your workout time. You should set aside a specific time each day for your exercise routine and make it a priority. This will help you stay consistent with your workouts and make them a part of your daily routine.

Break Up Your Workouts:

If you have a busy schedule, it can be challenging to find time for long workouts. Instead, try breaking up your workouts into shorter sessions throughout the day. For example, you can do 10-15 minutes of exercise in the morning, at lunchtime, and in the evening. This will help you stay active and burn calories throughout the day.

Make Use of Your Commute:

If you commute to work, you can use this time to incorporate physical activity into your routine. You can walk or bike to work instead of driving or taking public transportation. This will help you burn calories and stay active, even if you have a busy day ahead.

Choose Activities You Enjoy:

Incorporating physical activity into your routine is much easier if you choose activities you enjoy. This could be anything from dancing, hiking, swimming, or even gardening. When you enjoy what you are doing, you are more likely to stick with it and make it a part of your daily routine.

Make it a Family Affair:

If you have a family, you can make physical activity a family affair. You can take walks or bike rides together, go on hiking trips, or even participate in sports together. This will not only help you stay active but also provide quality time with your loved ones.

Use Technology:

There are many fitness apps and wearable devices available that can help you track your physical activity and monitor your progress. You can use these tools to set goals, track your progress, and stay motivated.

Prioritize Sleep:

Getting enough sleep is essential for weight loss and overall health. When you are sleep-deprived, you are more likely to skip workouts and make unhealthy food choices. Make sure to prioritize sleep and aim for at least seven hours of sleep each night.

In conclusion, incorporating physical activity into your busy lifestyle is essential for effective weight loss and maintaining a healthy weight. By scheduling your workouts, breaking them up into shorter sessions, making use of your commute, choosing activities you enjoy, making it a family affair, using technology, and prioritizing sleep, you can successfully incorporate physical activity into your routine and achieve your weight loss goals. Remember to start small and gradually increase your activity level to avoid burnout and injury.

## Strategies for Incorporating Physical Activity into Your Busy Lifestyle

Incorporating physical activity into a busy lifestyle can be challenging, but it is crucial for maintaining overall health and wellness. Regular exercise can improve cardiovascular health, reduce the risk of chronic diseases, and help manage stress and anxiety. Here are some strategies for incorporating physical activity into your busy lifestyle:

Schedule your workouts: Set aside specific times during the week for physical activity and schedule it into your calendar. This could be before work, during lunch breaks, or after work. By making a commitment to yourself and setting aside time for exercise, you are more likely to follow through with it.

Find an activity you enjoy: If you enjoy the activity you are doing, you are more likely to stick with it. Try different forms of exercise until you find something you enjoy, whether it be running, yoga, swimming, or hiking. This will make it easier to incorporate physical activity into your daily routine.

Make use of your lunch break: Use your lunch break to take a brisk walk or go to the gym. This is a great way to get some exercise during the day without sacrificing your work responsibilities.

Use active transportation: Instead of driving or taking public transportation, consider biking, walking, or running to work or other destinations. This will not only incorporate physical activity into your day, but it will also save money on transportation costs.

Take breaks and move around: Sitting for extended periods of time can be detrimental to your health. Take breaks throughout the day to stretch or take a short walk. This will help increase blood flow and energy levels.

Involve friends or family: Exercise can be more enjoyable when you do it with others. Involve your friends or family in your exercise routine, whether it be going for a walk or taking a fitness class together.

Make use of technology: There are many apps and wearable devices available that can help track your physical activity and provide motivation. Use these tools to set goals, track progress, and stay accountable.

Prioritize your health: It is essential to make physical activity a priority in your life. Make sure to take care of your body and make time for exercise, even on the busiest of days. Your health and well-being should always come first.

In conclusion, incorporating physical activity into a busy lifestyle is possible with proper planning and commitment. By finding an activity you enjoy, making use of your lunch break, taking breaks throughout the day, involving friends and family, and using technology, you can make exercise a regular part of your routine. Prioritizing your health and making time for physical activity is crucial for maintaining overall health and wellness.

Tracking Your Progress" on Lose Weight and Stay Busy: Tips for Effective Weight Loss

When it comes to losing weight, one of the most important things you can do is track your progress. Not only will this help you stay motivated, but it will also allow you to make adjustments to your plan as needed. Here are some tips for effectively tracking your progress:

Use a food diary: Write down everything you eat and drink throughout the day. This will help you identify areas where you can make healthier choices and where you may be consuming too many calories.

Weigh yourself regularly: Weigh yourself once a week or every other week to track your progress. This will give you a sense of how much weight you're losing and how quickly.

Take measurements: In addition to weighing yourself, take measurements of your waist, hips, thighs, and arms. This will help you see changes in your body composition, even if the scale doesn't budge.

Keep a workout log: Write down your workouts and the amount of weight you're lifting or the number of reps you're doing. This will help you see improvements in your strength and endurance over time.

Use technology: There are many apps and websites that can help you track your progress, from calorie counting apps to fitness trackers. Find one that works for you and use it consistently.

Set goals: Set realistic goals for yourself and track your progress towards them. This will help you stay motivated and focused on your weight loss journey.

Remember, tracking your progress is not about being perfect or hitting all your goals every time. It's about staying mindful of your choices and making adjustments as needed to reach your ultimate goal of losing weight and staying healthy.

## Planning Your Meals and Snacks for Maximum Weight Loss

Planning your meals and snacks is an essential part of maximizing your weight loss efforts. When you have a plan in place, you can ensure that you're eating a balanced diet and avoiding unhealthy choices that can sabotage your progress. Here are some tips for planning your meals and snacks for maximum weight loss:

Create a meal plan: Take some time each week to plan out your meals for the week ahead. This will help you stay organized and ensure that you have healthy, nutritious meals on hand.

Focus on whole foods: Choose whole, unprocessed foods as much as possible. These foods are typically lower in calories and higher in nutrients, which can help you lose weight while still feeling satisfied.

Balance your macronutrients: Make sure your meals contain a balance of protein, healthy fats, and complex carbohydrates.

This balance will help you feel full and satisfied while providing the nutrients your body needs to function properly.

Incorporate fiber: Choose high-fiber foods like fruits, vegetables, and whole grains. Fiber can help you feel full and satisfied, while also promoting healthy digestion.

Plan your snacks: Plan healthy snacks to keep you fueled throughout the day. This can help prevent overeating at meals and keep your energy levels stable.

Cook at home: When possible, cook your meals at home. This will give you more control over the ingredients and help you avoid unhealthy additives and preservatives.

Don't skip meals: Skipping meals can actually slow down your metabolism and make it harder to lose weight. Make sure you're eating regular meals and snacks throughout the day.

Remember, planning your meals and snacks doesn't have to be complicated. Focus on whole, nutritious foods and make sure you're getting a balance of macronutrients. With a little bit of planning, you can set yourself up for success on your weight loss journey.

## Making Positive changes to Lose Weight and Stay Busy: Tips for Effective Weight Loss"

Losing weight and staying busy can be challenging tasks for many people. However, it is essential to prioritize both aspects of your life for a healthier and happier lifestyle. Here are some tips for effective weight loss and staying busy:

Start with small changes: Making drastic changes to your diet and lifestyle can be overwhelming and unsustainable. Instead, start with small changes such as cutting down on sugar and processed foods or taking a 10-minute walk every day. Gradually, you can increase the intensity and duration of your activities.

Set realistic goals: Setting achievable goals can help you stay motivated and on track. Instead of aiming to lose 20 pounds in a month, set a goal to lose 1-2 pounds a week. This can be achieved through a combination of healthy eating and regular exercise.

Keep track of your progress: Monitoring your progress can help you identify what works and what doesn't. Keep a food diary, track your workouts, and take progress photos to see how far you've come.

Find an activity you enjoy: Exercise doesn't have to be a chore. Find an activity that you enjoy, such as dancing, hiking, or swimming, and incorporate it into your routine. This will make it easier to stick to your exercise plan.

Make healthy eating a habit: Eating healthy doesn't have to be complicated or expensive. Focus on incorporating more fruits, vegetables, whole grains, and lean proteins into your diet. Avoid processed foods, sugary drinks, and excessive snacking.

Stay hydrated: Drinking enough water is essential for weight loss and overall health. Aim to drink at least eight glasses of water a day.

Get enough sleep: Lack of sleep can lead to overeating and weight gain. Aim to get 7-9 hours of sleep every night to help your body recover and stay energized.

Find a support system: Losing weight can be challenging, but having a support system can make all the difference. Find a workout buddy, join a support group, or talk to friends and family about your goals.

In summary, losing weight and staying busy requires dedication and effort, but it is achievable. By making small changes, setting realistic goals, finding activities you enjoy, eating healthy, staying hydrated, getting enough sleep, and finding a support system, you can reach your weight loss goals and maintain a healthy and active lifestyle.

Mindful Eating: Tips for Staying Focused and Avoiding Distractions Lose Weight and Stay Busy: Tips for Effective Weight Loss"

Mindful eating is a practice that involves being present and aware of what you eat, how you eat it, and how it makes you feel. It can help you make healthier food choices, avoid overeating, and enjoy your meals more fully. Here are some tips for staying focused and avoiding distractions while practicing mindful eating:

Eliminate distractions: When you're eating, eliminate any distractions such as watching TV, scrolling through your phone, or reading. By focusing solely on your meal, you can tune into your hunger and fullness cues.

Chew your food: Chewing your food thoroughly can help you slow down and enjoy your meal more fully. It also aids in digestion and can prevent overeating.

Take small bites: Taking small bites and savoring each one can help you appreciate the flavors and textures of your food. It can also help you eat more slowly and feel more satisfied with your meal.

Use your senses: Use your senses to fully experience your meal. Notice the aroma, texture, and flavor of your food. Take time to appreciate the colors and shapes of the ingredients on your plate.

Pause between bites: Take a moment to pause between bites and check in with your hunger and fullness cues. This can help you avoid overeating and tune into your body's needs.

Practice gratitude: Before you start eating, take a moment to express gratitude for your food and the effort that went into preparing it. This can help you appreciate your meal more fully and be more mindful while eating.

Be aware of emotional eating: Mindful eating can also help you identify and address emotional eating. When you're tempted to eat out of boredom, stress, or sadness, take a moment to pause and check in with your emotions. Practice self-care and find healthier ways to cope with your feelings.

In summary, mindful eating is a powerful tool for making healthier food choices, enjoying your meals more fully, and avoiding overeating. By eliminating distractions, chewing your food, taking small bites, using your senses, pausing between bites, practicing gratitude, and being aware of emotional eating, you can Stay focused and be more mindful while eating.

Tracking Your Progress: Tools and Techniques for Measuring Success on Lose Weight and Stay Busy: Tips for Effective Weight Loss"

Losing weight and staying on track can be a challenging process, but tracking your progress can help you stay motivated and reach your goals. There are many tools and techniques available for measuring success when it comes to weight loss. Here are some tips and resources to help you stay on track and achieve your weight loss goals.

Use a food diary: Keeping a food diary can be a powerful tool for weight loss. By tracking what you eat, you can identify patterns and make changes to your diet that can help you reach your goals. There are many apps and websites available that can help you keep track of what you eat and provide insights into your eating habits.

Set achievable goals: Setting achievable goals can help you stay motivated and track your progress. When setting goals, be specific and realistic. For example, instead of setting a goal to lose 50 pounds, set a goal to lose 1-2 pounds per week.

Use a fitness tracker: Fitness trackers can help you monitor your physical activity and track your progress. These devices can track your steps, distance, calories burned, and other metrics that can help you stay on track with your fitness goals.

Take progress photos: Taking progress photos can be a great way to see how far you've come and stay motivated. Take photos of yourself at the beginning of your weight loss journey and then periodically throughout your journey to see how your body is changing.

Celebrate small successes: Celebrating small successes along the way can help you stay motivated and on track. For example, if you hit a milestone in your weight loss journey, treat yourself to a non-food reward, such as a new outfit or a massage.

Get support: Having support from friends and family can make a big difference when it comes to weight loss. Joining a support group or finding a workout buddy can help you stay accountable and motivated.

Track your progress regularly: Regularly tracking your progress can help you stay on track and make adjustments to your plan as needed. Set aside time each week to review your progress and make any necessary changes to your plan.

In conclusion, tracking your progress is essential for effective weight loss. By using tools such as food diaries, fitness trackers, and progress photos, setting achievable goals, celebrating small successes, and getting support, you can stay motivated and reach your weight loss goals. Remember to track your progress regularly and make adjustments to your plan as needed to achieve long-term success.

The Role of Sleep in Weight Loss: Tips for Getting Quality Rest to Lose Weight and Stay busy. Tips to effective weight loss

Sleep plays a crucial role in weight loss, as it impacts both your metabolism and your ability to make healthy choices throughout the day. When you are well-rested, you have more energy, better focus, and a stronger willpower to make healthy food choices and exercise regularly. In contrast, when you are sleep-deprived, your body produces more of the hormone ghrelin, which stimulates hunger, and less of the hormone leptin, which signals fullness, leading to overeating and weight gain. Additionally, lack of sleep can also lower your metabolism, making it harder to burn calories and lose weight.

Here are some tips for getting quality rest to aid in weight loss:

Stick to a sleep schedule: Go to bed and wake up at the same time every day, even on weekends. This will help regulate your body's internal clock and promote better sleep.

Create a sleep-friendly environment: Make sure your bedroom is cool, quiet, and dark. Use blackout curtains, earplugs, or a white noise machine if necessary.

Avoid caffeine and alcohol: These substances can disrupt your sleep cycle, so it's best to avoid them at least six hours before bedtime.

Establish a bedtime routine: Create a relaxing bedtime routine to wind down before sleep. This could include reading a book, taking a warm bath, or practicing yoga.

Limit screen time: Avoid using electronic devices, such as smartphones and tablets, before bed, as the blue light can interfere with sleep.

Exercise regularly: Regular exercise can improve sleep quality and promote weight loss. Aim for at least 30 minutes of moderate-intensity exercise most days of the week.

Eat a healthy diet: A balanced diet that includes whole foods, fruits, vegetables, lean protein, and healthy fats can Improve sleep quality and support weight loss.

In addition to quality sleep, here are some tips for effective weight loss:

Track your food intake: Keeping track of what you eat can help you identify areas where you can make healthier choices.

Stay hydrated: Drinking plenty of water can help keep you feeling full and aid in weight loss.

Eat mindfully: Focus on your food while you eat, and avoid distractions like TV or your phone. This can help you eat more slowly and savor your food, leading to better digestion and satisfaction.

Incorporate strength training: Building muscle can help boost your metabolism and aid in weight loss. Aim for two to three strength-training sessions per week.
Find support: Joining a support group or working with a personal trainer or nutritionist can help keep you accountable and motivated throughout your weight loss journey.
Overall, getting quality sleep and making healthy choices throughout the day are key to effective weight loss. By prioritizing your sleep and making lifestyle changes, you can achieve your weight loss goals and improve your overall health and well-being.

The Power of Protein on Lose weight and stay busy. Tips to effective weight loss

Protein is an essential nutrient that plays a vital role in weight loss and weight management. It is important for building and repairing tissues in the body, and it also helps to keep you feeling full and satisfied after meals, which can lead to reduced calorie intake and weight loss. Here are some tips on how to effectively use the power of protein to lose weight and stay busy.
Start your day with protein: Eating a protein-rich breakfast can help to curb hunger and reduce cravings throughout the day. Some great breakfast options include eggs, Greek yogurt, and protein smoothies.

Choose lean protein sources: Lean proteins such as chicken breast, fish, and tofu are low in calories and high in protein. They can help you feel full for longer periods of time and support your weight loss efforts.

Snack on protein: Snacking on protein-rich foods like nuts, seeds, and protein bars can help to keep you full between meals and prevent overeating.

Make protein the star of your meals: Try to make protein the main focus of your meals by including lean protein sources such as grilled chicken or fish, and pairing them with vegetables and healthy fats.

Plan ahead: Meal planning and preparation can help you stay on track with your weight loss goals. Make sure to include plenty of protein-rich foods in your meal plan and have healthy snacks on hand for when hunger strikes.

Be mindful of portion sizes: While protein is important for weight loss, it is important to be mindful of portion sizes. Eating too much protein can lead to excess calorie intake, which can hinder your weight loss efforts.

Stay active: Exercise is also an important component of weight loss. Regular physical activity can help to increase muscle mass and boost your metabolism, which can help you burn more calories throughout the day.

In conclusion, incorporating protein-rich foods into your diet can be an effective way to support your weight loss efforts. By making smart food choices, planning ahead, and staying active, you can achieve your weight loss goals and maintain a healthy lifestyle.

Building a Support System: Finding Accountability and Encouragement in Your Weight Loss Journey

Losing weight can be a challenging journey, and having a strong support system can make all the difference. Building a support system of people who can hold you accountable and provide encouragement can help you stay motivated and on track with your weight loss goals. Here are some tips on how to find accountability and encouragement in your weight loss journey.

Share Your Goals and Progress with Family and Friends

Let your family and friends know about your weight loss goals and progress. This will help them understand what you are trying to achieve and how they can support you. They can help you stay accountable by asking about your progress and encouraging you to keep going when things get tough.

Join a Weight Loss Group

Joining a weight loss group can be a great way to find accountability and encouragement. There are many different types of weight loss groups, such as online communities, support groups, and fitness classes. Look for a group that fits your needs and goals, and make an effort to participate regularly.

Hire a Personal Trainer

A personal trainer can provide personalized guidance and support as you work towards your weight loss goals. They can help you create a workout plan that is tailored to your needs, and they can hold you accountable for sticking to your plan.

Find a Weight Loss Buddy

Finding a weight loss buddy can provide a great source of accountability and encouragement. Look for someone who has similar goals and is committed to making healthy changes in their life. You can support each other by sharing your progress and providing motivation when needed.

Use Social Media

Social media can be a powerful tool for finding accountability and encouragement. Join weight loss communities on platforms like Facebook and Instagram, and share your progress with others. Seeing other people's success stories can provide inspiration and motivation to keep going.

In conclusion, building a support system can be a game-changer in your weight loss journey. Whether it's through family and friends, weight loss groups, personal trainers, weight loss buddies, or social media, having people who can hold you accountable and provide encouragement can make all the difference. Remember that the most important thing is to stay committed to your goals and never give up.


Overcoming Obstacles on the Road to Weight Loss"

Weight loss can be a challenging journey that often involves obstacles along the way. While it's important to stay focused on your goal and remain motivated, it's equally important to be prepared for the challenges that may arise. In this article, we'll explore some common obstacles people face on their weight loss journey and strategies for overcoming them.

Lack of motivation: One of the biggest obstacles people face when trying to lose weight is a lack of motivation. To overcome this, it's important to identify your reasons for wanting to lose weight. Whether it's to improve your health, feel more confident, or fit into your favorite clothes, reminding yourself of your goals can help keep you motivated. Additionally, finding a workout buddy or joining a support group can provide accountability and encouragement.

Unrealistic expectations: Many people set unrealistic goals for themselves, such as losing a significant amount of weight in a short amount of time. When they don't see results quickly, they may become discouraged and give up. To avoid this, it's important to set realistic goals and be patient. Remember, slow and steady progress is more sustainable than quick fixes.

Social pressure: Social pressure can be a major obstacle when trying to lose weight. Friends and family members may encourage you to indulge in unhealthy foods or skip workouts. To overcome this, it's important to communicate your goals and boundaries with your loved ones. Let them know that you're committed to making healthy choices and ask for their support.

Plateaus: Plateaus are a common obstacle that people face on their weight loss journey. They occur when your body adapts to your new routine and stops losing weight. To overcome a plateau, try mixing up your workout routine or changing your diet. Adding in strength training or increasing your protein intake can also help jumpstart weight loss.

Emotional eating: Many people turn to food for comfort when they're feeling stressed, anxious, or bored. This can sabotage weight loss efforts and lead to a cycle of emotional eating. To overcome this, it's important to find healthier ways to manage emotions, such as exercise, meditation, or talking to a therapist.

In conclusion, while there may be obstacles on the road to weight loss, there are also strategies for overcoming them. By setting realistic goals, finding motivation and support, and making healthy choices, you can achieve your weight loss goals and improve your overall health and wellbeing.

Celebrating Success: Rewards and Incentives for Meeting Your Goals on weight Loss

Losing weight is a challenging journey that requires discipline, commitment, and perseverance. It's not easy to change your lifestyle and eating habits, but with the right mindset and support, you can achieve your weight loss goals. One way to keep yourself motivated and on track is to celebrate your success with rewards and incentives.

Rewarding yourself for reaching your weight loss milestones can help you stay motivated and committed to your goals. The rewards don't have to be extravagant or expensive; they can be simple yet meaningful. For example, you can treat yourself to a new workout outfit, a relaxing massage, or a night out with friends. The key is to choose rewards that align with your values and interests and that make you feel proud of your progress.

In addition to rewards, you can also use incentives to stay on track with your weight loss goals. Incentives are like rewards, but they are tied to a specific behavior or action. For example, you can set a goal to lose a certain amount of weight within a specific timeframe, and if you reach that goal, you can give yourself an incentive, such as a weekend getaway or a new gadget you've been eyeing.

Here are some tips for creating effective rewards and incentives for weight loss:

Set specific goals: To create meaningful rewards and incentives, you need to have clear, specific goals. Instead of just saying you want to lose weight, set a specific target, such as losing 10 pounds in two months.

Make it challenging but achievable: Your goals should be challenging enough to keep you motivated, but also realistic enough to be achievable. Setting unrealistic goals can lead to frustration and disappointment.

Choose rewards that motivate you: Your rewards should be things that motivate you and make you feel good about your progress. If you're not a fan of shopping, a new outfit might not be the best reward for you.

Create a reward system: To keep yourself accountable, create a reward system that outlines the specific rewards you'll give yourself for reaching your goals. Write it down and keep it somewhere visible as a reminder of what you're working towards.

Don't rely solely on rewards and incentives: While rewards and incentives can be helpful, they shouldn't be the only thing motivating you. Remember why you started your weight loss journey and focus on the benefits of a healthy lifestyle.

In conclusion, celebrating your success with rewards and incentives can be a powerful motivator in achieving your weight loss goals. By setting specific, challenging but achievable goals and choosing rewards and incentives that motivate you, you can stay committed and on track towards a healthier lifestyle.

## The Changes: Adopting a Healthier Lifestyle on weight loss

Adopting a healthier lifestyle can lead to significant changes in weight loss. It is important to note that weight loss is not just about cutting calories and increasing physical activity. It is about making sustainable changes in your habits and behaviors to support a healthy lifestyle.

One of the most significant changes to adopt a healthier lifestyle is to focus on whole, nutrient-dense foods. This means choosing foods that are minimally processed and rich in vitamins, minerals, and fiber. Examples of these foods include fruits, vegetables, whole grains, lean proteins, and healthy fats. By focusing on these foods, you can increase satiety and decrease the likelihood of overeating.

Another important change is to increase physical activity. This can include structured exercise such as running, cycling, or weightlifting, as well as simple activities like walking, gardening, or taking the stairs instead of the elevator. Increasing physical activity not only burns calories but also has numerous health benefits such as reducing the risk of chronic diseases and improving mental health.

In addition to diet and exercise, other lifestyle changes can support weight loss. These include reducing stress, getting enough sleep, and limiting alcohol intake. Stress can lead to overeating or making poor food choices, so finding ways to manage stress such as through meditation or yoga can be helpful. Getting enough sleep is important for overall health and can also support weight loss by regulating hormones that control appetite and metabolism. Finally, limiting alcohol intake can reduce calorie intake and improve overall health.

It is important to remember that adopting a healthier lifestyle is a process that takes time and effort. It is not about quick fixes or fad diets but rather about making sustainable changes that you can stick with over the long term. By focusing on whole foods, increasing physical activity, and making other lifestyle changes, you can support weight loss and improve your overall health and well-being.

Achieving Healthier Life Goals on weight Loss

Achieving a healthier life goal of weight loss can be challenging, but it is definitely achievable with dedication and perseverance. Here are some tips to help you achieve your weight loss goals:

Set a Realistic Goal: The first step to achieving your weight loss goals is to set a realistic goal. It is important to set a goal that is achievable and not too far-fetched. For example, losing 1-2 pounds per week is a realistic and healthy goal.

Create a Plan: Once you have set your goal, it's time to create a plan. Your plan should include a healthy diet, regular exercise, and lifestyle changes. A well-planned diet that is rich in fruits, vegetables, whole grains, and lean proteins can help you lose weight in a healthy way. Also, incorporating regular exercise into your daily routine can boost your metabolism, help you burn calories and build muscle.

Keep Track of Your Progress: Keep a record of your progress. This can be done by keeping a food diary, tracking your weight loss, or monitoring your exercise routine. Keeping track of your progress can help you stay motivated and make necessary adjustments to your plan if needed.

Stay Motivated: Motivation is key to achieving your weight loss goals. Surround yourself with positive influences, such as friends or family members who support your goals. Find inspiration through success stories of people who have achieved their weight loss goals.

Be Patient: Losing weight is not an overnight process. It takes time and effort to achieve your goals. Be patient with yourself and do not give up if you do not see results immediately. Celebrate small successes along the way to keep yourself motivated.

In conclusion, achieving a healthier life goal of weight loss requires dedication, patience, and a well-planned approach. With the right mindset and a solid plan, you can achieve your weight loss goals and live a healthier and happier life.

## The Benefits of Healthy Lifestyle after losing weight

Losing weight can be an important step towards a healthier lifestyle, but it's not just about the number on the scale. Adopting healthy habits can have numerous benefits beyond weight loss. Here are some of the benefits of a healthy lifestyle after losing weight:

Improved overall health: Eating a nutritious diet and exercising regularly can reduce your risk of chronic diseases such as heart disease, diabetes, and certain cancers. Losing weight can also reduce the strain on your joints and improve your mobility.

Increased energy: When you're carrying excess weight, it can take a lot of energy just to move around. Losing weight and adopting a healthy lifestyle can help you feel more energized and able to tackle daily tasks more easily.

Better sleep: Poor sleep can lead to a host of health problems, including weight gain. By losing weight and adopting healthy habits, you may find that you sleep better, which can improve your mood, energy levels, and overall health.

Boosted confidence: Losing weight and feeling better about your body can boost your self-confidence and self-esteem. This can have a positive impact on all aspects of your life, from personal relationships to professional opportunities.

Improved mental health: Research suggests that adopting healthy habits such as regular exercise and a nutritious diet can have a positive impact on mental health. Losing weight and feeling better about your body can also help alleviate symptoms of depression and anxiety.

Better quality of life: By adopting a healthy lifestyle, you may find that you have more energy, better mobility, and improved overall health. This can lead to a better quality of life, allowing you to enjoy activities and experiences that you may have previously avoided.

In conclusion, losing weight and adopting healthy habits can have numerous benefits beyond just shedding pounds. By prioritizing your health and wellbeing, you can improve your overall quality of life and enjoy all the benefits that come with a healthy lifestyle.

Improved Health After Weight Loss

Weight loss can have numerous benefits for one's health, both physical and mental. Shedding excess pounds can lead to improvements in overall wellbeing, reduce the risk of various chronic diseases, and increase life expectancy.

One of the most significant benefits of weight loss is the reduction in the risk of developing chronic diseases such as type 2 diabetes, cardiovascular disease, and certain types of cancer. Being overweight or obese increases the risk of these diseases, and losing weight can help reduce that risk. Additionally, weight loss can improve existing conditions such as high blood pressure and high cholesterol, which can further reduce the risk of developing cardiovascular disease.
Weight loss can also have a positive impact on joint health. Carrying excess weight can

put a strain on joints, particularly the knees, hips, and back. By losing weight, the pressure on these joints is reduced, leading to less pain and better mobility.

Improved mental health is another benefit of weight loss. People who are overweight or obese are more likely to experience depression, anxiety, and low self-esteem. Weight loss can improve mood and self-confidence, leading to a more positive outlook on life.

Improved sleep is another benefit of weight loss. Sleep apnea, a condition in which breathing is disrupted during sleep, is more common in people who are overweight or obese. Losing weight can reduce the severity of sleep apnea and improve overall sleep quality.

In addition to the physical and mental benefits, weight loss can also lead to an improved quality of life. Simple activities such as walking, climbing stairs, and playing with children or grandchildren can become easier and more enjoyable. This can lead to a greater sense of independence and a more active lifestyle.

Overall, weight loss can have numerous positive effects on one's health and wellbeing. While the journey to weight loss may not be easy, the benefits are well worth the effort. Consult with a healthcare professional to determine the best approach to weight loss that fits your individual needs and goals.

## The Ongoing Journey of Health and Wellness after weight Loss therapy

Weight loss therapy can be a transformative experience for many individuals, providing a kickstart to a healthier lifestyle and a newfound sense of confidence. However, the journey to health and wellness does not end once the therapy is complete. In fact, it is an ongoing journey that requires dedication, commitment, and a willingness to make permanent changes to one's lifestyle.

One of the most important aspects of maintaining a healthy lifestyle after weight loss therapy is to continue with healthy eating habits. This means consuming a balanced diet that is rich in whole foods, such as fruits, vegetables, lean protein, and healthy fats. It is also essential to pay attention to portion sizes and to limit the consumption of processed foods and sugary drinks.

Physical activity is another key component of a healthy lifestyle. After weight loss therapy, it is important to continue incorporating regular exercise into one's daily routine. This can include activities such as strength training, cardio, yoga, and other forms of physical activity that one enjoys. Regular exercise not only helps maintain weight loss but also has numerous other health benefits, including reducing the risk of chronic diseases such as heart disease, diabetes, and certain types of cancer.

Another important aspect of maintaining health and wellness after weight loss therapy is to prioritize self-care. This can include getting enough sleep, practicing stress-reducing activities such as meditation or deep breathing, and engaging in activities that bring joy and fulfillment. Self-care is crucial for both physical and mental health and can help prevent relapse and maintain long-term success.

It is also essential to have a support system in place after weight loss therapy. This can include family, friends, support groups, or a healthcare provider. Having a supportive community can provide accountability, motivation, and encouragement on the journey towards health and wellness.

In conclusion, the journey towards health and wellness after weight loss therapy is ongoing and requires a commitment to making permanent lifestyle changes. By continuing to prioritize healthy eating habits, regular physical activity, self-care, and having a support system, individuals can maintain their weight loss and improve their overall health and well-being.